I0422692

OVARIAN SURGERY RECOVERY DIET

Complete Guide Unlocking The Secrets Of
Nutrition To Rapid Healing After Surgery
Success, Nourishing Meal Plans, Recipes, Tips
For Optimal Health Wellness)

DR. ALLAN FREDA

Contents

ABOUT THIS BOOK

Through a carefully chosen diet plan, readers will find a complete guide to getting the best recovery after surgery. This book is written especially for people who have had ovarian surgery and it contains very useful information about how important diet is for healing.

There is a lot of useful information on its pages, like healing recipes, carefully planned meals, and expert advice to help people stay healthy in the long run. The diet plan is made up of different parts that are all meant to help the body heal faster and with fewer problems.

The book goes into detail about how important it is to eat right after ovarian surgery, focusing on the nutrients and foods that can help the healing process go faster. Every part of the diet plan is based on solid scientific study, from the important vitamins and minerals to the good antioxidants and anti-inflammatory foods.

"Rejuvenate" also stresses how important it is to look at healing as a whole, taking into account not only physical but also emotional and mental health. By giving readers useful tips and encouraging ideas, the author helps them fully grasp how diet can be an important part of their general recovery and long-term health.

"Rejuvenate The Ovarian Surgery Recovery Diet" is a must-read for anyone who wants to get healthy, whether they are newly identified or want to speed up their recovery after surgery. It has actionable advice, tasty recipes, and expert insights to help you on your way.

THE BEGINNING

How to Understand Recovery from Ovarian Surgery

Having surgery on your ovaries can be a big event in your life, whether it's for a mild condition like an ovarian cyst or a cancerous disease like ovarian cancer. After these kinds of surgeries, you need to pay close attention to many parts of your health, and your food is one of the most important ones. This detailed guide goes into great detail about ovarian surgery recovery diets, looking at the different aspects of eating after surgery to help with the best healing and long-term health.

A Look at Ovarian Surgery

Ovarian surgery includes many different procedures that are done to treat problems with the ovaries. These include cystectomy (removing ovarian cysts), oophorectomy (removing one or both ovaries), salpingo-oophorectomy (removing both ovaries and fallopian tubes), and debulking surgery for ovarian cancer. Traditional open surgery or minimally invasive methods like laparoscopy or robotic-assisted surgery may be used for these surgeries, based on the type of condition, how bad it is, and the patient's overall health.

There are different things to think about and problems that could happen with each type of ovary surgery. For example, a cystectomy keeps the ovaries working, but an oophorectomy removes one or both ovaries, which can cause menopause if done before the normal menopause age. After a diagnosis of ovarian cancer or to lower the risk of getting it in people with a high family risk, a salpingo-oophorectomy may be suggested. As much of the tumor as possible is removed during surgery for ovarian cancer. Chemotherapy or other treatments are often given afterward.

How Important Diet Is for Recovery

What you eat is very important for getting better after ovary surgery. Good nutrition helps wounds heal, lowers the chance of complications after surgery, and improves health in general. The body needs extra nutrients to heal cells, fight inflammation, and get stronger after surgery. Also, some food choices can help with complaints like nausea, constipation, and tiredness that are common after surgery.

A Complete Guide to the Best Diet for After Surgery

Healing Recipes, Meal Plans, and Expert Tips for Long-Term Wellness for People Who Have Just Been Diagnosed

When planning your food after surgery, you need to think about more than just getting enough calories. A healthy diet should have a mix of macronutrients (like carbs, proteins, and fats) and micronutrients (like vitamins and minerals) that are needed for cells to work and the immune system to stay strong. Also, staying hydrated is very important for keeping blood flow steady, improving circulation, and getting rid of toxins.

Recipes for Healing

Adding healing foods to a person's diet after surgery can help them stay healthy while also meeting their specific nutritional needs and digestive concerns.

A lot of the time, these recipes focus on whole, barely processed foods that are high in vitamins, minerals, and phytonutrients. Smoothies made with leafy greens, fruits, nuts, and seeds are full of nutrients and can be used as a quick meal replacement. One dose of these smoothies provides water, fiber, and antioxidants. Soups and broths, especially those made with veggie stock or bone broth, are easy on the digestive system and give your body the electrolytes and amino acids it needs to heal.

Plans for meals

Structured meal plans can help people better manage their diet after surgery, making sure they get all the nutrients they need while also taking into account any dietary limits or preferences.

A healthy meal plan usually includes a range of foods from different food groups, spread out over several meals and snacks during the day. It's important to eat a lot of fruits and vegetables, healthy fats (like avocado, olive oil, and nuts), lean proteins (like chicken, fish, and tofu), and complex carbohydrates (like whole grains, legumes, and starchy veggies).

To keep people from eating too much and help them feel full, portion control and careful eating may also be used.

Tips from experts for long-term health

In addition to eating well right after surgery, making healthy habits a part of your everyday life can help you stay healthy and have better surgical outcomes in the long run. Depending on your abilities and level of recovery, regular physical exercise can help you keep your muscle mass, improve your circulation, boost your mood, and make your life better in general. Rest and sleep are both very important for helping the body heal and fix parts that were damaged during surgery.

Mindfulness meditation, deep breathing exercises, and doing fun things in your free time are all good ways to deal with stress and improve your mental health.

Follow-up care with surgeons, dietitians, and other experts is also important to make sure that recovery is going well, that any problems or concerns are dealt with, and that dietary and lifestyle suggestions are changed as needed. Support groups, counseling services, and survivorship programs can be very helpful for people who are going through treatment for ovarian cancer. They can give them mental support, useful information, and a sense of empowerment throughout their journey.

the time after ovary surgery when a person is recovering is a very important part of their healing process. People can improve their health, speed up their recovery, and enjoy a better quality of life after surgery by putting nutrition first, eating a balanced diet full of healing foods, sticking to organized meal plans, and using expert advice for long-term wellness.

Disclaimer

The information in this book is for informational purposes only and should not replace professional medical advice, diagnosis, or treatment. Always consult your physician or a qualified health provider regarding any medical concerns. Do not disregard professional medical advice or delay seeking it based on information in this book.

The author does not endorse or have affiliations with any mentioned entities. References are for informational purposes only.

Consult your healthcare provider before making dietary or lifestyle changes, especially during recovery from surgery, as individual needs vary.

Results may vary, and the information provided is not guaranteed to produce specific outcomes.

By reading this book, you acknowledge and agree to consult your healthcare provider before implementing any information herein.

For further guidance, consult your healthcare provider or reputable medical websites for reliable information on surgery recovery diets.

CHAPTER 1
GETTING READY FOR RECOVERY

Before getting into the details of an ovarian surgery recovery diet, it's important to know how important it is to get ready for the journey ahead. Surgery of any kind can be hard on the body and needs a lot of rest, good nutrition, and a supportive setting to heal properly. Getting ready for healing includes setting up your kitchen, stocking it with the things you'll need, and learning how to plan meals so that you can easily start eating normally again after surgery.

Getting your kitchen ready:

Setting up your kitchen to meet your food needs is one of the first things you should do to make sure you have a quick and easy recovery from ovarian surgery. To do this, you need to set up your kitchen so that healthy foods and cooking tools are easy to get to.

You might want to rearrange your fridge and pantry to make room for healthy foods like fresh fruits and veggies, lean proteins, whole grains, and healthy fats. Getting rid of processed and bad-for-you snacks can also help you stick to your healing diet.

Additionally, make sure that your kitchen has all the necessary tools and appliances to make making meals easy, especially in the early stages of recovery when your energy may be low.

You should buy a good blender for making soups and drinks, a food processor for chopping and pureeing food, and cookware that is easy to use and clean. Having these tools on hand can make making healthy meals faster and easier without requiring too much effort.

Stocking Up on Important Ingredients:

During the recovery time, it's important to keep your kitchen stocked with the foods you need to eat a healthy, well-balanced diet. Focus on eating a wide range of nutrient-dense foods that will help you heal and stay healthy in general. Some important things to keep in your fridge and pantry are

1. Fresh fruits and vegetables: Choose a wide range of colorful fruits and vegetables that are high in antioxidants, minerals, and vitamins. Leafy greens, berries, citrus fruits, carrots, and bell peppers are all great foods that can help your body heal and reduce inflammation.

2. Lean proteins: To help repair tissues and muscles, eat lean forms of protein like chicken, fish, tofu, beans, and eggs. Protein is very important for treating wounds and getting stronger after surgery.

3. Whole grains: Eating whole grains like brown rice, quinoa, oats, and whole wheat pasta will give

you long-lasting energy and important nutrients like minerals, fiber, and B vitamins.

Whole grains can also help keep blood sugar levels in check and make you feel full.

4. Healthy fats: Eat foods like avocados, nuts, seeds, olive oil, and fatty fish like salmon and mackerel that are high in healthy fats. These fats are very important for getting fat-soluble vitamins, lowering inflammation, and keeping the brain healthy.

5. dairy products or dairy alternatives with added calcium and vitamin D: Choose low-fat dairy products or dairy alternatives with added calcium and vitamin D to help your bones stay healthy and your immune system works well. You could choose healthy foods like Greek yogurt, almond milk, or cheese made from skim milk.

6. Herbs and spices: Turmeric, ginger, garlic, cinnamon, and basil are some herbs and spices that can make your food taste better. These

ingredients not only give food more flavor, but they may also be good for you because they have anti-inflammatory and antioxidant qualities.

How to Plan Your Meals:

Planning meals well is important for keeping a healthy, well-balanced diet while you're recovering. Making plans ahead of time can help you feel less stressed, save you time, and make sure you have healthy meals on hand when you're tired. Here are some ideas to help you plan your meals:

1. Plan your meals ahead of time: Take the time to plan your meals for the week, taking into account your dietary needs, preferences, and any special dietary restrictions or advice from your healthcare provider. Making a planned meal plan ahead of time can help you avoid making bad choices at the last minute and promote better eating habits.

2. Make a lot of meals at once and freeze them. For example, make a lot of soups, stews, casseroles, and grain salads that can be frozen and eaten later.

This way, you can always have a range of home-cooked meals ready to go that only need a little work to reheat and serve.

3. Variety is important. To make sure you're getting all the nutrients you need, try to include a wide range of foods in your meal plan. If you want to keep meals interesting and fun, try using different foods, flavors, and ingredients.

4. Include a lot of fluids: To stay hydrated, drink a lot of water, herbal teas, broths, and freshly made juices throughout the day. Staying hydrated is important for helping the body heal, improving circulation, and getting rid of toxins.

5. Listen to your body. Notice when you're hungry or full, and listen to what it wants while you're recovering. Aim for balanced meals that include a

mix of carbs, protein, and healthy fats. Eat when you're hungry and stop when you're full.

You can make the most of your time recovering from ovarian surgery by getting your kitchen ready, making sure you have all the goods you need and smartly planning your meals.

Putting nutrition and self-care at the top of your list of priorities can help you heal, improve your general health, and support your long-term health and vitality.

CHAPTER 2
FOODS THAT HEAL TO RECOVERY

Diet is a very important part of getting better after ovarian surgery because it helps the body heal, lowers inflammation, and supports general health. A well-planned diet after surgery can help you heal faster, avoid problems, and have better long-term health. This detailed guide goes into detail about the idea of the best diet after surgery, focused on foods that are high in nutrients, low in inflammation, and good for your immune system to help you get better.

Ingredients High in Nutrients

To support tissue repair, immune function, and overall health, recovery from surgery requires a lot of important nutrients. Adding foods that are high in nutrients to your diet is very important for reaching these goals.

Vitamins, minerals, and antioxidants are all found in large amounts in fresh fruits and veggies.

All of these are important for healing and lowering the risk of getting infections. There are a lot of vitamins A, C, and K in leafy greens like spinach, kale, and Swiss chard. They also have minerals like iron and calcium that are important for bone health and muscle repair.

Lean proteins are also very important for healing after surgery because they provide the building blocks needed for muscle and tissue repair. Including lean protein sources in your diet, like chicken, fish, tofu, beans, and low-fat dairy, can help your body heal faster. Also, eating whole carbs like oats, quinoa, and brown rice gives you steady energy and important nutrients like fiber, B vitamins, and minerals, which help your body heal and keep your digestive system healthy.

Including healthy fats in your diet can also help you recover from surgery.

Salmon, flaxseeds, and walnuts are all high in omega-3 fatty acids, which are anti-inflammatory foods that can help reduce swelling and speed up healing. Other great foods that are high in healthy fats that are good for you and help you recover are avocados, olive oil, and nuts.

Foods That Reduce Inflammation

When the body is hurt or traumatized, including during surgery, it naturally reacts with inflammation. However, too much inflammation can slow down the mending process and make recovery take longer. So, adding anti-inflammatory foods to your diet after surgery is very important for controlling inflammation and helping your body heal properly.

Turmeric, a spice known for its anti-inflammatory effects thanks to its active compound curcumin, can be used in many dishes or taken as a supplement to help reduce inflammation and speed up the healing process.

Ginger is another strong anti-inflammatory that can be used to help digestion and lower inflammation after surgery. It can be added to teas or meals.

Also, eating a lot of different colored fruits and veggies can help fight inflammation because they are full of antioxidants and phytochemicals. Tomatoes, berries, cherries, and oranges all have a lot of vitamin C and other antioxidants that fight free radicals and lower inflammation. Cruciferous veggies like broccoli, Brussels sprouts, and cauliflower have a chemical called sulforaphane in them. This chemical has strong anti-inflammatory properties that can help people recover from surgery.

Also, adding plants and spices like rosemary, cinnamon, and garlic to food not only makes it taste better but also reduces inflammation, which helps the body heal. People can reduce inflammation, ease pain, and speed up the healing process by putting anti-inflammatory foods at the top of their post-surgery diet list.

It is very important to boost the immune system after ovary surgery to avoid getting infections or other problems that could slow down the healing process. Eating foods that boost the immune system can strengthen the body's defences and improve health in general.

Vitamin C is found in large amounts in citrus fruits like oranges, lemons, and grapefruits. Vitamin C is a powerful antioxidant that helps the immune system work by increasing the production of white blood cells and making it easier for the body to fight off illnesses. Kiwi, oranges, and bell peppers are also great sources of vitamin C that can be added to the diet after surgery to help the immune system.

Foods that are high in probiotics, like yogurt, kefir, cabbage, and kimchi, have good bacteria that help keep your gut healthy and your immune system strong.

A good balance of gut microbiota is important for keeping the immune system in check and protecting against pathogens. These probiotics help keep that balance.

Zinc-rich foods, such as lean meats, fish, nuts, and seeds, can also help the immune system work better and speed up the healing of wounds. Zinc is important for healing after surgery because it helps the immune system do many things, like making immune cells and controlling inflammatory reactions.

During the recovery time, adding immune-boosting herbs and spices like echinacea, elderberry, and astragalus to teas or meals can also help the immune system work better and improve overall health. By focusing on immune-boosting foods, people can boost their defences, lower their risk of getting infections, and speed up the healing process after ovary surgery.

the best way to use food to help with healing after surgery is to focus on foods that are high in nutrients, reduce inflammation, and boost immunity. By following these guidelines during the post-surgery diet, people can help their bodies heal, reduce inflammation, and boost their immune systems, which will lead to long-term health and an easier healing process.

CHAPTER 3

BREAKFASTS TO FUEL YOUR BODY

To get better after ovarian surgery, you need to pay close attention to your food and nutrition. The time after surgery is very important for healing, and eating the right foods can help a lot with that by speeding up the healing process, lowering inflammation, and giving you important nutrients. This is a complete guide to the best diet after surgery for people who have just been diagnosed.

It covers many parts of nutrition and includes meal plans, healing recipes, and expert advice for long-term health.

Many people think that breakfast is the most important meal of the day because it affects your energy and health in general. After ovary surgery, it's important to start the day with healthy foods that give you energy and help your body heal. Here are some breakfast choices that are good for helping you recover:

Getting energized smoothies

Smoothies are a great choice for breakfast, especially as you heal from surgery and may find it hard or painful to chew. They are simple to process, full of nutrients, and can be changed to fit each person's tastes and dietary needs. If you want to make a drink that gives you energy, start with leafy greens like spinach or kale.

These are full of vitamins and minerals. Berries, bananas, and mangoes are good foods to add sweetness and extra nutrients. To help your muscles heal and fix, try adding protein sources like Greek yogurt, tofu, or protein powder to your diet. You can also add healthy fats from things like nuts or avocado to your smoothie to make it even healthier. If you want, you can add water, coconut water, almond milk, or dairy milk to the blender and blend it all together until it is smooth and creamy. Energizing smoothies are a great way to start the day because they are both delicious and healthy.

Protein is an important part of your diet after surgery because it helps your body heal and keeps your defense system strong. You can easily and personally add protein-rich foods to your breakfast bowl, which makes it very handy. Put together a base of whole grains like oats, quinoa, or brown rice. These give you complex carbs and fiber that will make you feel full. Then add low-fat proteins like tofu, eggs, grilled chicken, or smoked salmon. For extra nutrients and fiber, you can add different kinds of veggies, like roasted sweet potatoes, sautéed spinach, or avocado slices. For extra flavor and health benefits, sprinkle your breakfast bowl with healthy fats like olive oil or tahini and herbs and spices.

Breakfast bowls that are high in protein are a tasty and filling way to help your body heal after ovary surgery.

Muesli and porridge that heal

Muesli and muesli are great choices for breakfast because they are warm and comfortable. This is especially true while you are recovering and may want foods that make you feel better. Oats are healthy whole grains that are high in fiber, vitamins, and minerals like magnesium, phosphorus, and manganese.

Muesli or muesli that is good for you can be made by cooking muesli with water, milk, or dairy-free milk like almond milk or coconut milk. Spices like cinnamon, vanilla powder, or mashed banana can be used to add flavour and nutrients.

Add Greek yogurt, chia seeds, or nut butter to get extra protein. Fruits like apples, berries, or dried figs can also be added for sweetness and extra nutrients.

Healing porridges and muesli are easy on the stomach and full of nutrients that help with healing and health in general.

Adding these healthy breakfast choices to your diet after surgery can help you heal, give you more energy, and improve your health in the long run. Try mixing and matching different flavors and ingredients to find mixtures that you like and that meet your dietary needs. Don't forget to pay attention to how different things make you feel and listen to your body. You can speed up your healing after ovarian surgery and set yourself up for a full and happy life by putting nutrition first and making healthy choices.

CHAPTER 4
SOUPS AND BREAD THAT ARE GOOD FOR YOU

Soups and broths that are good for you can help people who have recently had ovary surgery feel better. These liquid-based meals help the body heal by giving it calories, water, and warmth. They are also easy on the digestive system. Let's take a closer look at the idea of Wholesome Soups and Broths to see what they mean for meals after surgery.

Comforting vegetable broths are an important part of the diet for recovering from surgery because they provide the minerals, vitamins, and water that the body needs to heal. To make a tasty and healthy broth, people often use vegetables like celery, onions, garlic, carrots, and potatoes. There are a lot of vitamins in these foods, which help reduce swelling and speed up the healing of tissues. In addition, the warmth of veggie broth can help the body feel better after surgery, making it easier to get nutrients while reducing pain.

During the recovery process, it's important to eat a variety of soups that are high in protein to help rebuild tissues and keep your general strength up. Adding protein sources like lean chicken, turkey, tofu, or legumes to soups helps muscles and tissues heal by adding important amino acids. Soups that are high in protein can also help keep muscle strength, stop muscle loss, and boost the immune system. Getting protein from a range of sources helps you get enough and heal faster after surgery.

Healing bone broths are highly valued for their powerful healing effects and nutritional value, which makes them a great addition to a diet for recovering from surgery. Animal bones and connective parts are simmered for a long time to make bone broth. This releases nutrients like collagen, gelatin, amino acids, and minerals.

These nutrients help the body heal by supporting healthy gut bacteria, healthy joints, and flexible skin. Regularly drinking bone broth can also help reduce swelling, improve digestion, and boost immune system function, all of which are good for your general health while you heal.

Adding Wholesome Soups and Broths to a diet for recovery after surgery needs careful thought about the ingredients and how they are made to get the most nutrition and help the body heal. People can make sure they get the most health benefits from healing foods by choosing nutrient-dense ingredients like veggies, lean proteins, and bones from organic and grass-fed sources. Incorporating herbs, spices, and seasonings can also improve the taste of food while also offering health benefits like reducing inflammation and killing germs.

To make a complete guide to the best diet after surgery, you need to pay close attention to every detail and think about each person's needs, tastes, and dietary restrictions.

This book with healing recipes, meal plans, and expert advice makes sure that people can find a wide range of healthy foods that will help them on their way to recovery. People can confidently get through the recovery period after surgery if they have the right information and tools. This will help them heal better and stay healthy in the long run.

CHAPTER 5
HEALTHY SALADS AND SIDES

Salads and side dishes are an important part of any recovery diet, but they are especially important after ovarian surgery because they give you important nutrients, help your body heal, and improve your general health. After surgery, eating fresh, tasty salads, nutrient-dense side dishes, and healing grain and bean salads can help you get better faster and improve your health and well-being in the long run.

Fresh salads with lots of flavor:

Fresh, tasty salads are a great addition to any diet after surgery because they are full of vitamins, minerals, antioxidants, and plants that help the body heal and fight off illness. Most of the time, these salads have a wide range of healthy foods in them, like fruits, herbs, nuts, leafy greens, and colorful veggies.

Adding leafy greens like spinach, kale, or arugula and colorful veggies like bell peppers, tomatoes, cucumbers, and carrots to your salads can make them taste better and be better for you.

Aside from that, adding fruits like sliced apples, berries, or citrus fruits can add more vitamins and antioxidants, and herbs like basil, cilantro, or parsley can make it taste better and help reduce inflammation.

Nuts and seeds like almonds, walnuts, pumpkin seeds, and sunflower seeds can be added to foods to make them more filling and add texture. They also contain healthy fats, protein, and fiber.

If you make your sauces with olive oil, vinegar, lemon juice, and herbs instead of buying them, you can avoid the added sugars and preservatives that are often in store-bought dressings and still get the nutrients and flavor you need.

Side dishes that are high in nutrients are important for a person who has recently had surgery because they provide a concentrated number of vitamins, minerals, protein, and fiber that help the body heal and recover. Many of these side dishes have a mix of whole grains, legumes, root veggies, and leafy greens. This gives your body a healthy mix of macronutrients and micronutrients to help it heal.

Adding whole grains like quinoa, brown rice, farro, or barley to side meals can give you complex carbs, fiber, and important nutrients like magnesium and B vitamins, which your body needs to make energy and heal itself.

Also, adding legumes like chickpeas, edamame, lentils, or black beans can give you a plant-based source of protein, fiber, and micronutrients like iron and folate, which can help your muscles heal and your immune system work better. Root veggies, such as beets, carrots, sweet potatoes, and parsnips, can make side dishes sweeter and more filling.

They are also a great way to get a lot of vitamins, minerals, and antioxidants. Greens like Swiss chard, collard greens, and bok choy can be added to side meals to make them healthier and higher in nutrients. They can also help reduce inflammation.

Using healthy cooking methods like steaming, roasting, or sautéing with little to no extra fat can also keep the nutrients of the ingredients while making the food taste and feel better. Herbs, spices, and seasonings can also be used to give side dishes more depth and variety without adding too much salt or unhealthy fats. Overall, choosing side foods that are high in nutrients can help you eat better after surgery and help your body heal and recover.

Healthy Salads with Grains and Beans:

Healing grain and legume salads are flexible and healthy choices that can be eaten as main dishes or as side dishes.

They contain the right amount of carbs, protein, fiber, and other nutrients to help the body heal and recover after ovarian surgery.

A base of cooked grains or legumes is often used in these salads, which are then filled with different veggies, herbs, nuts, seeds, and dressings to make them taste, feel, and be healthy.

Adding whole grains like couscous, quinoa, bulgur wheat, or wild rice to grain salads can make the base filling healthy, with complex carbs, fiber, and important vitamins and minerals. Also, cooked legumes like chickpeas, black beans, kidney beans, or lentils can be added to salads to add protein, fiber, and vitamins like iron and folate, which help the body heal muscles and keep its immune system strong.

Adding different colorful vegetables like bell peppers, cucumbers, red onions, cherry tomatoes, and shredded carrots can also make grain and bean salads look better and be healthier by adding vitamins, minerals, antioxidants, and phytonutrients. Nuts and seeds, like almonds, sunflower seeds, pumpkin seeds, or hemp seeds, can add crunch, texture, and healthy fats.

Fresh herbs, like parsley, cilantro, mint, or basil, can add flavor, taste, and other health benefits.

Adding homemade vinaigrettes made from olive oil, vinegar, lemon juice, Dijon mustard, and herbs to grain and legume salads can add flavor and moisture without adding too many unhealthy fats or sugars, making sure you eat a healthy and enjoyable meal. Avocado, hummus, or Greek yogurt can also be added to salads to make them creamier and richer while also increasing the protein and healthy fat content. Overall, healing grain and legume salads are a handy and healthy choice for people who have had ovarian surgery because they provide important nutrients and improve overall health and vitality.

CHAPTER 6
FINISHING THE MAIN COURSES

When someone has ovarian surgery, they need to make sure they eat right to help them recover and stay healthy overall. Full-flavored main dishes are very important for giving the body the nutrients it needs to heal properly. There should be a good mix of lean proteins, plant-based options, and healing one-pot meals in these major courses.

Choices for lean protein

As the body's building blocks, proteins are very important during the healing phase after surgery. Lean protein options are low in fat and easy to digest, which makes them great for people who have recently had ovary surgery. Skinless chicken or turkey breast, lean cuts of beef or pork, fish, tofu, tempeh, and low-fat dairy products like yogurt or cottage cheese are all good sources of lean protein. These high-protein foods give your body the important amino acids it needs to repair tissues and build muscle without adding extra cholesterol or saturated fats. Adding lean protein options to main courses makes sure that patients get the nutrients they need to heal without putting their general health at risk.

Protein dishes made from plants

Adding plant-based protein dishes to your meals after surgery can be very helpful for people who are on a veggie or vegan diet or who just like plant-based foods. Plant-based proteins are a great source of nutrients and also have important vitamins, minerals, and enzymes that help the body heal and fight off illness.

Legumes (like black beans, chickpeas, and lentils), soybeans, quinoa, tofu, tempeh, nuts, seeds, and some whole grains (like farro or barley) are all great plant-based sources of protein. These protein-rich plant foods can be used in a lot of different main dishes, like salads, stir-fries, soups, and grain bowls. This gives patients a lot of different, tasty choices to help them get better.

One-Pot Meals That Heal

One-pot meals are simple, quick, and often very healthy, which makes them a great choice for people who are recovering from ovarian surgery. These meals usually have protein, carbs, and veggies all in one dish. This way, you don't have to cook and clean up as much, but you still get a healthy, filling meal. Soups, stews, casseroles, and skillet meals are all examples of healing one-pot meals that can be changed to fit each person's dietary needs and tastes. Adding healthy foods like lean proteins, whole grains, colorful veggies, herbs, and spices that help the body heal can make these meals more nutritious and help people get better faster. Making bigger amounts of one-pot meals ahead of time also makes sure that patients have easy access to healthy meals while they are recovering, which lowers their stress and keeps them fed while they focus on healing.

the main dishes that fill you up are important parts of a diet for recovering from ovarian surgery. Including lean protein choices, plant-based protein dishes, and healing one-pot meals in meals helps make sure that patients get the nutrients they need to heal, stay healthy, and have a successful long-term recovery. People can speed up their healing and improve their quality of life after surgery by focusing on nutrient-dense foods and adding a range of flavors and textures to their main courses.

CHAPTER 7
DRINKS AND FOODS THAT MAKE YOU FEEL BETTER

It is important to focus on a recovery diet that helps with healing, gives you more energy, and supports your general health after ovarian surgery.

One important part of this diet is drinking drinks that are soothing and that help you stay hydrated and healthy. Drinking these drinks can help a lot with pain relief, reducing swelling, and speeding up the body's healing process.

Herbal teas to help you relax:

People know that herbal teas can help you relax and calm down, which makes them a great choice for people who are healing from ovarian surgery.

For example, apigenin and other compounds found in chamomile tea have been shown to have anti-inflammatory and antioxidant qualities.

Chamomile tea is also known for having mild calming effects that can help reduce stress and improve the quality of sleep, both of which are important for healing.

Peppermint tea is another good plant tea that is loved for its soothing effects and ability to ease digestive problems. Peppermint has menthol in it, which is a natural substance known for its pain-relieving and muscle-spasmodic properties.

 This makes it especially good for getting rid of bloating or stomach pain after surgery.

Additionally, ginger tea is liked for its ability to reduce inflammation and help with nausea, which can happen after surgery because of anesthesia or painkillers. Bioactive substances in ginger, such as gingerol and school, can help reduce inflammation and soothe the digestive system. This makes ginger a great choice for recovering from surgery.

Adding these herbal drinks to your diet after surgery can help with both your physical and mental comfort by helping you relax, digest food better, and feel better overall while you're healing.

Elixirs and infusions that heal:

People who have had ovarian surgery can benefit from healing infusions and elixirs as well as plant teas. Often, these drinks have a mix of healing ingredients that are high in nutrients and give the body a powerful boost as it tries to fix itself.

Turmeric golden milk is an example of a healing beverage. It has turmeric, which is a strong anti-inflammatory spice, warm milk, and other healing spices like ginger and cinnamon. Curcumin, a bioactive compound found in turmeric, has strong anti-inflammatory and antioxidant qualities that can help reduce swelling and pain after surgery and speed up the healing of tissues.

Bone soup is another well-known healing liquid. It is full of minerals, amino acids, and collagen, all of which are important for repairing and growing new tissues.

Bone broth can help the body make more collagen, keep the gut healthy, and boost the immune system, all of which are important for a full recovery after surgery.

Adaptogenic herbs, such as ashwagandha or holy basil, can also be added to healing infusions to help lower stress, support adrenal function, and boost general resilience while the body heals.

These plants have been used for hundreds of years in traditional medicine because they help with balance and health. This makes them helpful on the road to recovery after surgery.

By adding healing infusions and elixirs to the recovery diet, people can give their bodies the nutrients and support they need to heal properly and stay healthy in the long run.

Drinks that hydrate and nourish:

Staying hydrated is very important for healing after surgery because it helps cells work, gets rid of waste, and keeps the body's fluid balance in check.

To support general health and well-being, it is important to include drinks that are both hydrating and nutritious in the recovery diet.

Plain water, which is important for staying hydrated and supporting body processes, is one of the easiest and most effective drinks for keeping you hydrated. Getting enough water throughout the day can help the body get rid of toxins, keep it from getting dehydrated, and heal itself naturally.

Coconut water is another great drink that keeps you hydrated and gives you electrolytes like magnesium and potassium, which are important for keeping your fluid balance and helping your muscles work. Coconut water also has cytokinins in it, which are plant hormones that are antioxidants and may help lower inflammation and speed up tissue repair.

Adding fresh veggie juices to the recovery diet can also help because they contain a lot of vitamins, minerals, and antioxidants that help the body heal and nourish cells. To get the most health benefits from these juices, choose veggies that are high in nutrients, like kale, spinach, carrots, and beets.

In addition, adding protein-rich smoothies or shakes to the healing diet can help muscles heal and rebuild, especially for people who may have lost muscle mass or become weak after surgery. Adding Greek yogurt, protein powder, leafy veggies, and healthy fats like avocado or nuts can help make a drink that is both filling and good for you. It can also help your body heal and recover overall.

People can support their bodies' natural healing processes, replenish important nutrients, and promote long-term health and vitality by making drinking nourishing beverages a priority and a part of their post-surgery diet.

CHAPTER 8

TREATS TO INDULGE IN

While recovering from ovarian surgery, it can be fun to eat desserts, but it's important to pick foods that help with healing and general health.

During the healing process, desserts can make you feel good and give you a sense of comfort.

They should also meet your body's nutritional needs and help it heal. In this part, we'll talk about healthy desserts, fruit-based treats, and healing dessert smoothies that can help you eat better after surgery while still satisfying your sweet tooth.

Desserts that are full of nutrients

After ovarian surgery, it's important to eat desserts that are high in nutrients to help the body recover and get its energy back. These desserts are full of vitamins, minerals, and antioxidants that your body needs to repair cells and keep your immune system strong. Desserts with nuts, seeds, whole grains, and dark chocolate are better for you because they contain many nutrients and are good for you. A homemade granola bar made with oats, nuts, seeds, and dried fruits is a sweet treat that is also good for you because it has fiber, protein, and healthy fats. In the same way, chia seed pudding with fresh berries and honey on top is both tasty and good for you. It has omega-3 fatty acids, fiber, and vitamins. You can enjoy sweets without hurting your health or healing if you pick desserts that are high in nutrients.

Fruit-based sweets

Fruit-based sweets are a great way to satisfy your sweet tooth while also giving your body the vitamins, minerals, and fiber it needs. Berries, apples, bananas, and citrus fruits are all fresh foods that are naturally sweet and good for you in many ways. Adding these fruits to sweets can make them taste and feel better while also making them healthier.

Fruit bowls, fruit skewers, or fruit parfaits with yogurt and granola are some ideas. If you want a more decadent treat, grill some fruit, like bananas or peaches, and serve them with some Greek yogurt and cinnamon on top. You can also make smoothie bowls that are both healthy and refreshing by blending frozen fruits with a splash of coconut water or almond milk. Not only do fruit-based sweets satisfy your sweet tooth, but they also help your body heal and improve your general health after surgery.

Fruit smoothies for health

Healing treat smoothies are a tasty and easy way to get the nutrients your body needs while also helping it heal and recover. These drinks are full of ingredients that are known to reduce inflammation, fight free radicals, and boost the immune system. This makes them perfect for nutrition after surgery. When you make a salad, start with leafy greens like spinach or kale. These are full of minerals and vitamins A, C, and K.

Berries, pineapple, or mango are good foods to add for sweetness and extra vitamins and antioxidants. Add things like Greek yogurt, almond butter, or protein powder to increase the amount of protein you eat and help tissues heal. You can also add healing spices like ginger or turmeric, which can help with pain control and recovery because they reduce inflammation. Add any drink you like, like almond milk, coconut water, or herbal tea, and blend it all together until it's smooth and creamy. After ovarian surgery, healing dessert smoothies are a tasty way to feed your body and help it heal properly.

CHAPTER 9
SNACKS TO KEEP YOU GOING

Keeping up your energy during the recovery time after ovarian surgery is very important for helping your body heal and improving your overall health. It's important to eat snacks because they give you the nutrients and energy your body needs to heal properly. Adding a range of snacks to your diet after surgery can help keep your blood sugar stable, help your body heal, and keep you from getting tired. This article talks about three types of snacks that can help you stay energetic and get better: nut and seed mixes, healing fruit and vegetable snacks, and protein-packed snack ideas.

Mixed nuts and seeds

Nut and seed mixes are easy to make and full of nutrients for people who have had ovary surgery. There are a lot of good fats, protein, fiber, vitamins, and minerals in these snacks. All of these things help the body heal itself. Almonds, walnuts, peanuts, pumpkin seeds, sunflower seeds, and chia seeds may all be in a healthy mix. One food that is high in vitamin E is almonds. Vitamin E is an antioxidant that helps reduce inflammation. Omega-3 fatty acids, which are found in walnuts, are good for your heart and may help ease pain after surgery.

Cashews are a good source of magnesium, which is important for nerve and muscle activity. Pumpkin seeds have a lot of zinc, which helps the defense system work and heal wounds. Sunflower seeds have selenium and vitamin E, which are good for your skin and nervous system. Chia seeds have a lot of fiber, which is good for your gut system and makes you feel full. By mixing these nuts and seeds, you get a powerful mix of nutrients that can keep you going all day. Making these mixes into single amounts makes it easy to get a quick and healthy snack while you're recovering.

Adding healthy fruit and veggie snacks to your diet after surgery gives you the vitamins, minerals, antioxidants, and fiber you need to help your body heal and stay healthy overall. Fruits and veggies are full of nutrients that help reduce swelling, boost the immune system, and speed up the healing of damaged tissues.

Choose a range of colorful fruits and veggies to get a wide range of nutrients. Berries like blackberries, raspberries, strawberries, and blueberries are full of antioxidants like vitamin C and flavonoids that help fight oxidative stress and fix cells. Citrus foods, like oranges, grapefruits, and lemons, contain vitamin C, which is needed to make collagen and keep your immune system healthy.

Also, citrus foods may help your body absorb iron, which is important for getting your iron stores back up after surgery. Leafy greens like spinach, kale, and Swiss chard are full of vitamins A, C, and

K, folate, and magnesium. These nutrients help keep your immune system healthy and help tissues grow back. Bell pepper, carrots, cucumbers, and celery are some other healing veggies that are high in vitamins, minerals, and phytonutrients. Adding these healthy fruits and vegetables to snacks like fruit salads, vegetable crudités with hummus, or shakes makes them a tasty and nutrient-dense way to help your body heal and keep your energy up.

Snack Ideas Packed Full of Protein

During the recovery time after ovarian surgery, it is important to eat snacks that are high in protein to help repair damaged tissues, keep muscle mass, and stop muscle loss. Getting enough protein in your snacks can help you feel full, keep your blood sugar stable, and speed up the healing process. Choose protein foods that are low in fat, like chicken, fish, tofu, tempeh, beans, eggs, and dairy. For instance, Greek yogurt has a lot of protein and probiotics, which are good for your gut health and immune system.

Cottage cheese is a quick and easy snack that can be used in many different ways. It has a lot of protein and calcium, which is good for your bones. Hard-boiled eggs are easy to carry and are full of nutrients like protein, vitamins, and minerals that your body needs to heal. Chickpea hummus has both protein and fiber, which helps you feel full and keeps your digestive system healthy.

Protein-rich snacks like turkey or chicken roll-ups with whole-grain wraps, tuna salad lettuce wraps, or edamame beans sprinkled with sea salt are a healthy and filling way to keep your energy up and help your body heal after surgery. Adding protein powder to smoothies or making your energy balls is another way to get more protein and help your body heal. Focus on getting protein from a range of sources to make sure you get enough of the essential amino acids your body needs to repair tissues and stay healthy in general.

snacks are very important for keeping up your energy and making it easier to heal after ovary surgery. Nut and seed mixes, healthy fruit and veggie snacks, and snack ideas that are high in protein are all good ways to give the body the nutrients it needs at this very important time. By eating a variety of snacks after surgery, you can make sure you get enough of the vitamins, minerals, antioxidants, and protein that your body needs to heal, reduce inflammation, and support your general health. After ovarian surgery, people can speed up their healing and improve their long-term health by making nutrient-dense snacks a priority and drinking plenty of water.

CHAPTER 10
TIPS AND SPECIAL THINGS TO THINK ABOUT

Following a well-planned and nutritious diet is very important for the healing process after ovary surgery. To heal quickly, control inflammation, and get stronger again, the body needs the right foods. Also, changes to the diet may be needed to meet special needs that came up after surgery and to keep the person healthy while they recover. Along with what you eat, making sure the kitchen is safe and practicing self-care are also important parts of a holistic approach to healing after surgery.

Changes to the diet for certain needs

Depending on the type of surgery, the person's health, and any conditions they already had, they may have different dietary needs and problems after ovarian surgery. One example is that people who have had laparoscopic surgery may have less pain afterward and heal faster than people who have had open surgery. As a result, these groups may need different changes to their diets.

1. Soft foods that are easy to digest: In the days after surgery, people may feel sick, vomit, or have trouble swallowing because of the effects of the anesthesia or pain medicine. So, choosing soft foods that are easy to digest, like soups, broths, yogurt, and cooked veggies, can help reduce pain and make sure you get enough nutrients.

2. Fiber-Rich Foods: Constipation is typical after surgery, especially because of the anesthesia, painkillers, and decreased physical activity. Eating fiber-rich foods like fruits, veggies, whole grains, and legumes can help with constipation and make it easier to go to the toilet regularly. But it's important to add fiber slowly so that you don't have any stomach problems.

3. Foods High in Protein: Protein is an important part of the diet after surgery because it helps repair tissues and heal wounds. Lean protein sources like chicken, fish, eggs, tofu, and legumes can help the body recover and keep muscles from losing mass when you don't do as much physical exercise.

4. Hydration: Staying hydrated is important for healing after surgery because it helps keep the body's fluid balance, supports cell function, and makes it easier for the body to get rid of toxins. To stay healthy and avoid getting dehydrated, drink a lot of water, herbal teas, and other clear fluids throughout the day.

5. Vitamin and Mineral Supplements: Depending on the person's needs and food limits, vitamins and mineral supplements may be suggested to help them heal and avoid not getting enough of certain nutrients. Iron (to avoid anemia), calcium (for bone health), and vitamin D (for immune function and bone health) are common

supplements given to people who have had surgery.

Making sure the kitchen is safe during the recovery period is important to avoid accidents and lower the risk of harm, especially for people who may have trouble moving around, feel weak, or get dizzy after surgery. Putting these cooking safety tips into action can help make the area safer for making food:

1. Organise your kitchen: Keep tools, cookware, and items that you use often close at hand so that you don't have to bend, reach, or stretch as much. Think about changing the layout of your kitchen to make it easier to use and more comfortable.

2. Use Kitchen Gadgets and Tools: To keep your hands and arms from getting sore, use kitchen gadgets and tools like jar openers, electric can openers, and ergonomic utensils. Also, buy tools like slow cookers, rice cookers, and microwave

ovens to make cooking meals easier and cut down on the time it takes to do so.

3. To keep your kitchen floors safe from slips, trips, and falls, keep them clean, dry, and free of trash. Place mats or rugs that don't slip under sinks, stoves, and work areas to make them more stable and lower the risk of accidents.

4. Use safe cooking methods: To keep from getting burned while cooking, use oven mitts or potholders to hold hot pots and pans. Watch out for knives and other cooking tools that are very sharp, and be careful when you use them to avoid getting hurt.

5. Get Help: If you can, ask family, friends, or carers to help you make meals, go grocery shopping, and do other things around the house. Having a support system in place can help reduce stress and make sure that food needs are met while you are healing.

Along with what you eat and how safe your kitchen is, taking care of yourself can help you recover quickly and improve your general health after ovarian surgery. Adding the following self-care tips to your routine after surgery can help you heal faster and enjoy life more:

1. rest: After surgery, give yourself plenty of time to rest and heal. Pay attention to your body's signals and put sleep, rest, and dealing with stress at the top of your list of priorities to help it heal.

2. Gentle Exercise: Depending on what your body can handle, do light workouts like walking, stretching, or low-impact sports. Gradually get more active based on how much energy you have and any advice your healthcare provider gives you.

3. Pain Management: Do what your doctor tells you to do to deal with pain and soreness after surgery. As directed, take your painkillers and use warm pads or ice packs as needed to ease pain and swelling.

4. Emotional Support: Surgery can be hard on the body and the mind, so it's important to get emotional support from friends, family, support groups, or mental health workers if you need it. Talking about your thoughts, fears, and feelings can help reduce stress and improve your mental health.

5. Follow-Up Care: Make sure you keep all of your follow-up visits with your doctor so they can check on your recovery and talk to you about any worries or problems that may come up. To make sure you heal properly, do what they say about how to take care of wounds, handle medications, and limit your activities.

a complete plan for recovering from ovarian surgery includes changes to your diet, safety precautions in the kitchen, and self-care habits that will help you heal quickly and stay healthy in the long run. By making sure their kitchen is safe, meeting their specific nutritional needs, and putting self-care tasks at the top of their list of priorities, people can help their bodies heal and improve their quality of life during and after recovery.

CONCLUSION

To fully recover from ovarian surgery, you need to take a comprehensive approach that includes not only medical care but also careful consideration of your food choices and general health habits. In this detailed guide, we've gone into great detail about how to eat properly after surgery, showing you how important your diet is to your recovery and giving you useful tips on how to heal faster with food.

Every step of getting ready for life after surgery has been carefully outlined, from making sure you have all the ingredients you need in your home to planning healthy meals. Eating foods that are high in nutrients, contain anti-inflammatory ingredients, and improve your immune system is a good way to start healing.

The variety of healing recipes included, from breakfasts that will wake you up to soups that will warm you up and healthy main courses, not only focus on nutrition but also meet the need for tasty and filling meals while you're recovering. These recipes make sure that eating is still a pleasure instead of a chore by including choices for every taste and diet.

In addition, the fact that there are soothing drinks, decadent desserts, and filling snacks shows how important holistic nutrition is for supporting both physical and mental health during the recovery time. Understanding that nutrition and general health are linked, these offerings are meant to provide both sustenance for the body and comfort for the soul.

Also, special considerations and expert tips are very helpful for making changes to your food, making sure your kitchen is safe, and putting yourself first while you're recovering. Using these ideas in daily life can give people the tools they need to speed up their healing process and set them up for long-term health after surgery.

At its core, this complete guide is a lighthouse of support and direction for people who are starting to heal after ovarian surgery. People can start a trip towards holistic wellness by embracing the power of good nutrition, healing recipes, and expert tips. One healthy meal at a time, they can regain their health and vitality.

www.ingramcontent.com/pod-product-compliance
Lightning Source LLC
Chambersburg PA
CBHW070316290526
45791CB00003B/1136